GARDEN STATE HOSPITAL

GARDEN STATE HOSPITAL

STORIES OF ADMISSION AND TREATMENT TURMOIL

DR. TAMER SABRY

ADJUNCT PROFESSOR
UNIVERSITY OF THE PEOPLE

Copyright © 2024 by Dr. Tamer Sabry

All rights reserved.

No part of this book may be reproduced in any form or by any electronic or mechanical means, including information storage and retrieval systems, without written permission from the author, except for the use of brief quotations in a book review.

To my son Karas Sabry and my wife Jakleein Jakleein Sabry

CONTENTS

Introduction ix

1. The Admission Process 1
2. Quality of Care 11
3. Cleaning Staff and Hygiene 21
4. Discrimination and Inclusivity 29
5. Systemic issues and improvement strategies 37

Afterword 47
Bibliography 51

INTRODUCTION

New Brunswick, New Jersey, is home to Garden State Hospital, a leading Roman Catholic healthcare facility on Easton Avenue. The hospital was started in 1907 and has grown from a 25-bed hospital to a complex healthcare system with 478 licensed beds (Garden State Healthcare System, n.d.). It is affiliated with Garden State Healthcare System, Inc., a non-profit healthcare system supported by the Roman Catholic Diocese of Metuchen. The hospital's mission indicates its focus on providing quality health services and commitment to the ethical and moral standards of the Catholic Church. With time, Garden State Hospital has developed a strong reputation for offering specialized services. The hospital is recognized as Specialty Acute Care Children's Hospital, Regional Perinatal Center, and Stroke Center. It is also a large clinical training site for Rutgers Biomedical and Health Sciences and has a clinical affiliation with the Children's Hospital of Philadelphia.

INTRODUCTION

Even though this hospital has a long experience and provides many services on its site, Garden State Hospital needs more clarity from patients. This is evident from the 3.7 rating given by users from the 561 Google reviews it has received so far. These reviews present a somewhat mixed overall picture, where while there are beautiful things said about how patient-care-oriented the hospital is, there are also highly negative things said about things like medical mistakes and systems problems. This diversity of the reviews shows that the hospital is complex and can be both strong and weak simultaneously. Such a split places Garden State Hospital among the most suitable candidates for a detailed examination of its functioning and attitudes toward patients.

This book focuses on the patient experiences at Garden State Hospital and provides detailed information about its functioning. Hence, the analysis of the eyewitness testimonies and critique presented in this book should give the reader a glimpse of the hospital's advantages and disadvantages. By engaging in this systematic analysis, we strive to address questions about the quality of care and patient safety that could be relevant to Garden State and other healthcare organizations that experience similar difficulties.

Some key positive aspects found at Garden State Hospital are a passion for serving the community, sophisticated equipment, and many focused service lines. However, patients' feedback reveals substantial deficiencies such as delayed appointments, lack of cohesion among staff members, improper invoicing systems, and malpractice cases. Therefore, by systematically illustrating these strengths and weaknesses, this book seeks to paint an accurate picture of the hospital. The intent is not harmful, but it is to offer constructive feedback that could be instrumental in improving existing systems and patient experience in healthcare facilities.

In this book, the author divides the content into chapters dedicated to the hospital's functioning and patients' interactions. The first chapter, "The Admission Process," focuses on the earliest interactions between the patients and the hospital: admission logistics struggles with documentation and patient stories of these experiences. This chapter is intended to give a clear vision of the first stages of the patient experience to build a foundation for further analysis of this process.

The second chapter, Quality of Care, explores the medical knowledge of the employees, patients' outcomes, and the quality of doctor-patient interactions. To provide a balanced and comprehensive overview of the medical care at Garden State Hospital, this chapter will focus on several real-life cases, both positive and negative. It identifies factors that led to patient satisfaction and dissatisfaction, how the hospital has performed well, and how it has performed dismally.

The third chapter is about 'The Cleaning Staff and Hygiene,' which describes the cleaning staff, how clean the hospital is, and its effects on patients. In this chapter, the author seeks to draw attention to the role of cleanliness in a healthcare setting by evaluating patients' positive and negative remarks on the facility's cleanliness. It emphasizes the importance of cleanliness in contributing to the patient's healing process and satisfaction.

The fourth chapter, "Discrimination and Inclusivity," addresses reports on discrimination based on race, economic status, or disability. This chapter focuses on analyzing the extant policies implemented at the hospital to foster patient diversity and evaluate their success by using patient feedback. In this chapter, the author sought to share the successes and the failures of the hospital's attempts to make everyone feel welcome and treated well when seeking treatment.

The last chapter, "Systemic Issues and Improvement Strategies," discusses common systemic problems concerning the reviews, like management problems and lack of communication. It describes hospitals' role in patient trust and satisfaction and how it can be enhanced. Based on examples of other hospitals, this chapter attempts to share solutions that can help Garden State Hospital and other healthcare facilities overcome these systemic issues.

To this end, each chapter will be devoted to a particular analysis of one segment of the hospital's operation based on authentic patients' feedback and life stories. In this systemic manner, the book strives to present a fair perspective of Garden State Hospital to

INTRODUCTION

improve the general discussion concerning advancing healthcare quality and patient safety. This book aims to offer a comprehensive and complex analysis of the hospital to offer insights into enhancing the quality of healthcare services.

ONE
THE ADMISSION PROCESS

THE INITIAL ENCOUNTER

The patient's first impression of a hospital determines the rest of their experience with the health facility (Lindström et al., 2020; Liu et al., 2020; Marca-Frances et al., 2020). Admission at Garden State Hospital has received both positive and negative feedback from patients; some have been in a position to comment that the admission process was smooth with friendly admission staff, while others were complaining of delayed admission and other complicated procedures. Positive aspects are mainly related to the efficient organization of admission arrangements and the polite behavior of administrative personnel. Those patients admitted with smooth transitions enjoy the front desk officers' quick response and courtesy. For example, some account reviews praise the staff for their friendliness, especially during emergencies requiring rapid response.

These constructive interactions assist in establishing trust and confidence in the hospital to deliver quality healthcare.

However, not all patients feel this way about the service they are being provided with. Several have complained of long waits and many inconveniences in the admission process, especially where urgent treatment is needed. Some of the problems include increased patient anxiety and discomfort due to long waiting times. For instance, a patient shared an upsetting story in which they had to wait for 48-plus hours for an induction delivery appointment but had to be frustrated by mismanagement and lack of communication. This case points to one of the most sensitive issues, given that early admission plays a crucial role in managing a patient's condition. Such delays may adversely affect patient outcomes, especially for patients requiring prompt admission (Jones et al., 2022; Magnusson et al., 2020). Admissions need to be efficient to retain patients' trust and safety.

Further, some patients also complained of adverse experiences due to bureaucratic barriers. Form completion and confirmation of insurance information and medical records can be tedious and time-consuming. For patients with existing health problems, such additional administrative tasks can be stressful (Gagliardi et al.., 2021; Heinrich et al., 2022). Among common complaints, there are too many requests for the same data stemming from the need for more cooperation between various departments. A patient said they had to repeat their insurance details several times because the hospital could not keep records well, which exposed them to other hassles, such as billing.

These negative experiences underscore the need to reduce the admission cycle time so that patients get the right care at the right time. Despite the observed areas of competence in the hospital, the admission process has some areas that require enhancement. Solving these problems implies improving the cooperation between departments, eliminating unnecessary paperwork, and ensuring that all the staff involved in admissions are prepared to complete their work on time and efficiently. These changes can significantly benefit patient satisfaction and hospital organizational performance.

Overall, the first meeting with the organization through the Garden State Hospital admission process portrays contradicting experiences. Some patients have even had positive experiences characterized by efficiency and friendliness, while others have raised concerns such as long waiting times and bureaucratic procedures. Hence, the hospital should work to address these concerns and aim for a more efficient and patient-oriented admission process to improve the hospital's image and provide patients with a better beginning towards receiving the needed care (Prakash & Srivastava, 2020; Prakitsuwan & Promsit, 2022). The positive and negative comments are important for scrutiny as they point to areas of concern and underscore the importance of ongoing endeavors toward excellence in delivering health services.

DOCUMENTATION AND RED TAPE

Many patients face several challenges when handling the paperwork and bureaucratic system of Garden State Hospital. The main one is that the patient must complete a lot of paperwork at admission. Outpatients must tell about their previous illnesses, check their insurance details, and sign various consent forms. This official requirement constitutes an additional load for those who have chronic health problems. Due to multiple and cumbersome documentation, it becomes easier to commit mistakes, and a lot of time is spent on admissions procedures and access to healthcare as needed. The numerous and often elaborate documents can be overwhelming, resulting in mistakes and missing information, making the admission process more challenging and prolonging access to required medical attention (Rodziewicz & Hipskind, 2020; Singh et al., 2024). It is imperative to address these challenges to improve the experience of the patients and the timely access to services.

Delayed billing and insurance problems are also among the key concerns that Garden State Hospital patients face. This common problem is evident in most reviews, where patients are charged or billed for services that were never rendered. This is compounded by the fact that the hospital has done little to address these issues and their resolution. For instance, patients always complain that they receive the wrong bills that must be corrected due to clerical mistakes or communication misunderstandings. One patient provided an anecdote of a billing concern for a year. Even after the patients kept repeating their insurance information, the hospital seemed to lose the details every time, which caused many billing issues for the patients.

This is compounded by the fact that billing and documentation are not coordinated between hospital departments. It becomes a cycle of redundancy where patients have to start the process of explaining their symptoms and medical history all over again and again to different departments of the hospital. Further, the absence of such a process leads to time wastage and enhances the probability of developing faults in the system (Åhlin et al., 2022; Zepeda-Lugo et al., 2020). Another patient mentioned how they had to provide their insurance details several times to the hospital because the latter failed to update their records properly. This constant demand for the same documents points to a crucial area that requires enhancement to facilitate effective administrative functioning.

Such administrative issues can greatly affect the patient experience, as mentioned below. Thus, billing issues and complicated paperwork can create stress and confusion and negatively perceive the hospital (Ferreira et al., 2023). Additionally, billing concerns can pose a fiscal concern to patients since they may pay out-of-pocket despite having insurance (Kalouguina & Wagner, 2020). These issues are worsened by poor communication and poor follow-ups from the hospital; patients feel abandoned most of the time.

Evaluating record-keeping methods and other administrative procedures at Garden State Hospital can positively impact patient satisfaction and healthcare organization. It could be adopting improved methods in data management to minimize duplication, educating staff on how to handle documents correctly, or policies to deal with billing issues efficiently (Bhati et al., 2023; Mahmoudi et al., 2020; Verma et al., 2021). In this way, the hospital can minimize the time spent on paperwork by patients, and consequently, patients will spend more time on their treatment.

In conclusion, the documentation and bureaucracy at Garden State Hospital are burdens to the patients. Some of them are too much paperwork, problems concerning billing and insurance, and lack of cooperation between different departments. These issues raise concerns about the necessity of enhancing administrative structures to provide better patient experiences. Thus, by organizing documentation and focusing on follow-ups of billing-related matters, a particular hospital will become more effective and patient-satisfactory.

PATIENT NARRATIVES

Patients' stories offer valuable information about the actual consequences of the Garden State Hospital admission process. These personal stories explain the individual perspective of treatment providing and receiving, exposing both the pros and cons of the hospital's healthcare system. Studying these narratives will provide insight into the impact of administrative and operational issues on patients.

Another touching narrative is the one of a high-risk pregnancy appointment that was missed because the woman had to wait 25 minutes for an appointment. Given her condition, the patient was understandably stressed and frustrated when her appointment was canceled despite doing everything in an attempt to arrive on time. This cancellation was based on the fact that the hospital adhered strictly to a scheduled time without regard to the fact that this was a high-risk pregnancy. This lack of flexibility and understanding not only increased the patient's stress levels but also endangered her health and that of her unborn baby. Such experiences speak volumes of the need for hospitals to embrace higher levels of patient-centeredness when attending to patients with sensitive health complications.

One story was shared by a patient who had undergone his admission, where he experienced numerous delays and bureaucracy. They had all the documents and the insurance details; however, the patient was in a never-ending loop of requesting the same information. Every department was almost working independently, and there needed to be better communication between them, thus creating avoidable barriers. This made the patient feel frustrated and neglected, which affected their confidence in the hospital, especially in the timely provision of effective treatment. The patient's testimony underscores the need for integrated solutions and efficient communication channels across departments to improve patients' outcomes.

However, a few success stories show that, at least in some cases, Garden State Hospital can provide exceptionally satisfactory service. Several patients described how the admission personnel were extraordinarily polite and did everything they could to make the process seamless despite the high traffic. The excellent conduct of the staff, especially showing empathy when interacting with the patient, lifted his spirits and set the pace for the rest of his stay at the hospital. It is an excellent example of a story that illustrates the importance of a conscious and compassionate approach to patients' needs and their experiences.

However, even these positive narratives are steeped in the system's underlying elements that require change. For instance, a patient who was satisfied with the kindness of the nurses pointed out the issues with waiting for hours during admission. Such varied experiences reveal the paradoxical nature of patient care at Garden State Hospital, where quality can coexist with operational problems.

These problems need to be tackled systematically to enhance the admission process. This could include staff training, a more relaxed shift work approach, and improved organizational communication (Bhati et al., 2023; Damery et al., 2021). In those areas, Garden State Hospital can guarantee that all patients will have no stress and will only have positive impressions starting when they enter the premises.

In conclusion, patient narratives can help one understand the consequences of the admission process at Garden State Hospital. These stories emphasize the importance of integrated, adaptive, and patient-focused care to increase patient satisfaction. Notably, by tackling the challenges in these narratives, the hospital can go a long way in enhancing a positive healthcare delivery system.

TWO
QUALITY OF CARE

MEDICAL COMPETENCE AND PATIENT OUTCOMES

Garden State Hospital provides inconsistent care, as can be deduced from patients' ratings. On one hand, the majority of patients have reported that they have received professional and compassionate care in the hospital. These positive experiences are usually associated with the knowledge and hard work of the medical staff. For example, one of the patients shared his story of how he underwent a complicated surgery, and each surgeon and the nurse who treated him did a great job in the surgery and postoperative care. This patient also highlighted that the doctors were well-informed and ensured that the patient understood all the procedures, which helped reduce the anxiety level greatly. The nurses were caring and active in making the patient's recovery uneventful and comfortable. Such experiences raise the prospects of what is possible at Garden State, proving that the hospital can produce exemplary care when all the conditions are right.

However, the hospital has many negative reviews regarding medical care, including misdiagnosis and negligence, which led to the deterioration of patients' condition. One example relates to a traumatic labor and delivery process. The patient reported being left alone for hours on end with doctors giving out different information. The patient was described as high-risk, and the medical team did not communicate well. This resulted in a series of errors leading to an emergency C-section. Consequently, the patient said that the absence of communication and seeming disorganization among the staff not only exacerbated their physical pain but also traumatized them emotionally. This case underscores the significance of efficient communication and collaboration among the staff, with a special reference to the patient's safety during childbirth.

In other cases, patients have complained of misdiagnosis that resulted in additional operations and more suffering time. Another patient shared an experience when they received a wrong diagnosis and endured a long list of painful examinations and therapies. One has to go to another hospital to be referred to another doctor who corrects the diagnosis and discovers that all the previous treatments were doing more harm than good. This experience made the patient feel betrayed and lack confidence in the healthcare received at Garden State. Such incidents highlight the terrible consequences of diagnostic mistakes for the patient's condition and quality of life.

Still, many testimonies of patients saved due to treatment at Garden State Hospital. For example, one patient with a scarce and fast-growing type of cancer commended the oncology staff for knowledgeable and caring services. The patient narrated how the doctors came up with an individual treatment plan, which managed to bring the cancer into remission. The nurses were very supportive throughout the treatment process, ensuring the patient received physical and moral support. As elaborated in this story, the hospital can provide exceptional medical service, especially in complicated circumstances.

However, the mixed opinions indicate a major issue of the volatile quality of services delivered at Garden State Hospital. Some patients get the best care from the hospital,l while others receive poor care, affecting their confidence in the health facility. Solving these issues involves increasing communication, staff training, and adopting efficient quality assurance procedures (Buljac-Samardzic et al., 2020; Jankelová & Joniaková, 2021). By focusing on such aspects, the hospital can gradually guarantee the quality of care to all the patients they are owed.

Garden State Hospital's medical competence and patient results are nuanced. Although there are many success stories of professional and caring health care, there are also many complaints of medical malpractice and misdiagnosis. These two experiences underscore the importance of maintaining high quality and continuity of care across all departments. By addressing the precursors that result in adverse patient experiences, Garden State can improve its image and the destiny of all patients.

PATIENT-DOCTOR COMMUNICATION

Interpersonal communication between a patient and a doctor is an essential component that determines treatment returns (Drossman & Ruddy, 2020; Noble, 2020; Tavakoly Sany et al., 2020). In the case of patient experiences at Garden State Hospital, the quality of communication implicitly determines their level of trust and satisfaction. Effective communication means that the patients understand their conditions, treatment options, and prognosis, hence promoting their roles in their treatment. When doctors explain diseases and treatment options well, patients feel less anxious and actively participate in their treatment processes (Singh & Dey, 2021). Patients who get empathetic responses from the providers are likely to follow the recommended treatment plan and contribute their efforts towards recovery processes.

The communication between patients and doctors at Garden State Hospital indicates many positive instances. Many patients have reported that the medical staff is informative and less unresponsive. For example, one patient described how their doctor clearly explained the details of the illness and treatment. The doctor also took the time to respond to all the questions raised by the patient to make them feel comfortable with the treatment to be administered. Such a level of communication made the patient more comfortable with the situation and improved their confidence in the doctor. These are some of the best examples showing how important it is to communicate concisely and kindly with patients.

Nevertheless, only some patients seeking the services of Garden State Hospital have had such experiences. Concerning the communication breakdown, many reviews highlight patients being given different information from different physicians or inadequate information about their treatment. One of the most disturbing cases was a patient who was confused and anxious after receiving conflicting information from different specialists. The communication breakdown between the medical team made the patient uneasy about their diagnosis and unsure of what to expect next. This case exemplifies how improper communication undermines patient confidence and medical practice efficiency.

Some patients claimed the medical personnel did not acknowledge their concerns and symptoms. Such an attitude not only erodes the patient-physician rapport but also poses a threat to patient safety (Keshavarzi et al., 2022). In one of the interviews, a patient recounted how her symptoms were time and again dismissed by physicians, thus preventing a correct diagnosis and timely treatment. To worsen the patient's frustration and distress, there was an overwhelming sense that their voice was being ignored. Communication is informing the patient, listening, and considering the patient's opinion as part of the process. For instance, when patients are dismissed, it undermines their confidence in their doctors, which is not suitable for their health (Smith, 2017). It is important to address this issue to enhance patient satisfaction and overall health care.

Enhancing patient-doctor communication in Garden State Hospital can be complex. Doctors also benefit from communication skills training to communicate information in simple and compassionate ways (Boissy et al., 2016; Steinmair et al., 2022). Also, improving organizational culture regarding medical staff cooperation can minimize situations where patients receive contradictory information and increase the overall coherence of their treatment (De Brún et al., 2020). Standard operating procedures can also be adopted to guarantee that the patients receive accurate information regardless of the physician they encounter. Thus, by focusing on communication, the hospital can increase patient satisfaction and positively affect their health.

Overall, patient-doctor communication significantly predicts the quality of care at Garden State Hospital. As many positive examples of informative and qualified doctors exist, many problems are connected with confusion and a need for synchronization. Solving these problems is crucial for developing trust with the patient and achieving positive results in the treatment process. Therefore, by emphasizing effective interpersonal communication and teamwork, Garden State can improve its image and increase patient satisfaction across the spectrum.

CASE STUDIES

Interviews with individual patients allow for insight into the specific positive and negative aspects of Garden State Hospital, presenting a diverse picture of patient satisfaction. These case studies illustrate good practices and areas of neglect, providing a broad picture of the hospital's contribution to its patients.

A bright example is the case of a patient with impaired kidney function. During this patient's treatment process, they commended the hospital staff for the excellent treatment they received. On admission, they were attended to by competent nephrologists and professional nurses who were knowledgeable and caring. The doctors took their time to explain the patient's condition, the tests that needed to be carried out, and what would happen next. The patient was thus comforted and had faith in the medical team; their anxiety was significantly reduced. The nursing staff was friendly and attentive during the treatment process, constantly checking on the patient and asking if he needed anything. This case indicates the exceptional care possible at Garden State Hospital and how valuable it is to combine medical prowess with human warmth.

However, another anonymous patient's story shows significant deficiencies in-hospital treatment. This patient who was admitted to the hospital for a surgical procedure had a lot of negative experiences that could have been avoided. First, the patient mentioned that they had to wait for admission to the hospital for several days because of the mistakes that increased their stress before the surgery. The patient had a confused state of treatment because he received different information from different doctors during his stay. Inadequate coordination of the medical staff led to confusion and contradictory information being given to the patient regarding his treatment and recovery. Further, the patient felt abandoned as the nurses took time to attend to their needs. This story illustrates the areas that require the most focus at Garden State Hospital, mainly management and collaboration between departments.

One specific story belongs to a woman who experienced traumatic labor and delivery. This high-risk patient felt neglected during some of the most crucial points of her labor. They also reported that the medical team seldom and irregularly communicated their status to them, which was very distressing. There was a moment when the patient himself stated that he had severe pain and that there may be complications, but the staff did not pay attention to him for several hours. The absence of proper communication and what seemed to be chaos within the staff led to an emergency C-section, which the patient felt could have been prevented. This case emphasizes the risk of inadequate communication between patients and physicians and the general demand for enhanced attention to patients in critical medical states.

However, there would also be positive testimonies that show that it is still possible to receive excellent health care in this hospital. For instance, a patient with a particular type of cancer that is rare and considered aggressive narrated how the oncology staff at Garden State Hospital did not only offer medical care but also care beyond what was expected. The doctors devised the most appropriate working plan that best suited the patient's needs, and the nurses encouraged the patient throughout the treatment process. The patient's account suggests that the hospital can provide high-quality and comprehensive services, especially in complicated medical situations.

THREE
CLEANING STAFF AND HYGIENE

BEHIND THE SCENES: THE CLEANING CREW

The cleanliness department of Garden State Hospital is responsible for keeping the hospital clean and safe for the patients and employees. They are vital in ensuring that no infectious diseases are spread in the hospital and that there is overall compliance with health standards. The responsibilities of cleaning crews include cleaning and disinfecting patient rooms, equipment, and general cleanliness of the common areas. These procedures are sometimes unseen, yet invaluable for the hospital's functioning and the patient's condition.

The positive comments regarding Garden State Hospital's cleanliness indicate that the cleaning crew is hardworking and practical. Regarding cleanliness, many patients have commended the hospital for its good hygiene standards and the hardworking cleaning crews.

The patients said that their rooms are cleaned thoroughly every day, and they see the staff focusing on even the corners of the ward, the doorknob, and the rails of the bed. In addition to ensuring that the patient was comfortable during the recovery period, these measures also made the patient confident in the hospital's health and safety measures. One patient commented that the public areas, including the waiting areas and restrooms, were always clean, testifying to the professional conduct of cleaning services.

However, there are also bad reviews that can be attributed to issues in cleaning and maintenance. A few patients have also complained of dust and dirt in some hospital areas and questioned the facility's hygiene standards. The only complaints pointed out during the survey were the dust bunnies they found under the bed and dirty windowsills in their room. One patient described how shocked they were to find out that the floors were not clean and the restrooms were in bad shape during their stay. These negative reviews imply that despite many hardworking cleaning personnel, irregular cleaning procedures might require attention.

Hospital cleanliness is one of the most critical determinants of patients' health. HAIs have been identified as a major issue in hospitals, and cleaning and decontaminating surfaces are among the most important ways to avoid them (Haque et al., 2020). Maintaining proper hygiene in all corners of the hospital is extremely important to reduce the likelihood of HAIs and provide a protective environment for the patients and all the healthcare team members (Maki & Zervos, 2021). Hence, Garden State Hospital must mitigate any vulnerabilities in its cleaning practices that may compromise its sterilization standards.

Measures that could enhance cleaning reliability include: The hospital could conduct periodic training to inform the cleaning staff about the existing cleaning and infection control training. Also, planned checking and review of cleaning activities play a vital role in discovering factors that require enhancement and confirming compliance with excellent practices throughout the hospital (Flodgren et al., 2016). Therefore, by paying more attention to the cleaning personnel and enforcing proper cleaning measures, Garden State Hospital can improve cleanliness and patient satisfaction.

Overall, the cleaners at Garden State Hospital play a crucial role in ensuring that the hospitals are clean and infection-free. Although several reviews state that the staff members are doing their best, there are also complaints about the need for more hygiene that should be resolved. When proper attention is given to enhancing cleaning and standardization, the hospital offers a better environment to the patients and employees.

HYGIENE STANDARDS AND PRACTICES

Adequate hygiene is also important in hospitals to prevent infections among the patient and staff (Ahmad & Osei, 2023; van Hout et al., 2022). As with any healthcare facility, Garden State Hospital must employ strict

CLEANING STAFF AND HYGIENE

cleaning and disinfection procedures to reduce the likelihood of HAIs. They can complicate patients' conditions, resulting in longer hospital stays and higher medical expenses. Hygiene care measures include cleanliness of patient rooms and other areas, proper sanitation of clinical instruments, and strict observance of hand washing procedures by healthcare givers.

Patient feedback, which is typically positive, may include appreciation for the cleanliness and hygiene levels of Garden State Hospital. Those who speak positively often report that the cleanliness of the personnel and the room is exceptional. A patient testified that it was refreshing to observe that their hospital room was clean and well cared for during their stay. The second patient was also satisfied with the cleaning schedules and noticed that the staff was keen to disinfect frequently touched objects. These positive experiences suggest that the hospital has a clean environment, which is crucial for patient trust and safety.

However, some of the reviews include complaints about the lack of cleanliness, as well as poor maintenance of the hospital infrastructure. Some patients have complained of finding some parts of the hospital dirty or poorly maintained, and this causes them to doubt the general cleanliness of the hospital. For example, one of the patients could complain about the condition of the restrooms because they were not cleaned very often and lacked necessary supplies. One of the reviews also highlighted areas with dirt and dust in the patient's room, indicating that the cleaning procedures were not being adhered to. These negative accounts demonstrate that the hospital's hygiene is inconsistent and requires better supervision to enforce a high standard of hygiene across the facility.

There is ample evidence in the literature to support the need to observe high levels of hygiene to avoid getting infected. Peters et al. (2022) have noted that proper environmental cleaning and disinfection activities are significant strategies for preventing HAIs. The Centers for Disease Control and Prevention (CDC) also stresses the information of cleaning staff and adherence to the best practices to provide a safe healthcare environment. If the recommendations above are followed, then hospitals can reduce cases of HAIs and promote better outcomes for patients.

Garden State Hospital can improve its cleaning practices and conduct more frequent inspections and audits to address the variation in hygiene practices. It is crucial to guarantee that all employees, from cleaners to doctors, are educated about the measures necessary to prevent the spread of infections. Moreover, improving the quality of cleaning services using more advanced cleaning tools and products can contribute to higher cleanliness levels. Patient and staff feedback can also be sought periodically to determine areas that require change.

Therefore, it would be crucial for Garden State Hospital to adopt high hygiene practices to avoid potential infections that may be detrimental to the patient's health. While there are positive remarks concerning the hospital's hygiene in preparation for the disease, negative remarks indicate that more stringent measures need to be observed. By tackling these problems and conducting adequate cleaning, the hospital may improve its image and ensure a safe environment for everyone.

IMPACT ON PATIENT HEALTH

Hospital hygiene has a significant impact on the health of the patients as well as their recovery period. Maintaining hygiene is crucial since HAIs make the patient's condition worse and can cause severe health complications (Sharma et al., 2023). Hygiene manifested at Garden State Hospital through positive and negative accounts of the patient's health status. Proper sanitation creates a clean environment where patients do not easily fall sick or take a long time to heal. On the other hand, a lack of hygiene can cause discomfort, prolonged hospitalization, and other complications.

Success stories of patients at Garden State Hospital demonstrate the need for high standards of cleanliness. This has been supported by patients who have appreciated the effort made by the hospital to ensure the area is clean and free from bacteria/infections. For example, one surgery patient observed that the operating room and recovery area organization gave him confidence and comfort. Due to the assurance that the hospital could prevent infection, the patient was not anxious and could attend to the recovery process. Such experiences highlight hygiene's centrality in facilitating favorable conditions for healing and recovery.

However, there are also sad testimonies of patients who felt uncomfortable because of hygiene. One patient said he found his and other patients' soiled beddings and dirty floors in his room, as this worsened his anxiety and caused him discomfort throughout his stay. The non-wiping of surfaces and visible dirt and grime were a source of discomfort to them, besides the fear of getting infected. One patient complained about the rest facilities, observing that they found the restrooms dirty with overflowing bins and missing some necessities. Such circumstances were unhygienic and uncomfortable and did not contribute to the patient's well-being and healing process. They illustrate how poor hygiene's adverse effects affect patients' overall health in facilities they attend.

There is sufficient evidence to conclude the relationship between hospital cleanliness and the condition of patients in health facilities. Research has also established that better cleaning methods and strict hygiene measures can prevent HAIs (Asamrew et al., 2020). Healthcare workers' adherence to hand washing, environmental cleanliness, and proper cleaning and fumigation of patients' rooms are very important measures in preventing infections (Umuhoza & Amanyi, 2023). It is important to guarantee adherence to these practices to prevent patient deterioration and facilitate faster healing.

The patients' experiences at Garden State Hospital

show that more efforts should be devoted to enhancing hygiene. To prevent these issues, cleaning personnel should be trained frequently, the premises inspected often, and any inadequacies corrected as soon as possible. Patients' feedback can help analyze problem areas and find ways to deal with them (Han et al., 2023). When it comes to hygiene and addressing patients' concerns, the hospital's quality of services should improve, making the environment more safe for healing.

Therefore, cleanliness plays a significant role in health standards at Garden State Hospital. Whereas positive experiences focus on the positive social consequences of maintaining high standards of cleanliness, negative experiences show the possible pain and health consequences of low standards. The hospital must attend to these challenges and remind everyone to uphold high hygiene standards to promote patient well-being. Every patient must receive a clean, sanitary environment, promoting positive health and quick recovery.

FOUR
DISCRIMINATION AND INCLUSIVITY

PATIENT EXPERIENCES WITH DISCRIMINATION

Discrimination in health care setting can produce devastating and long-term effects on patients (Stangl et al., 2019; Togioka et al., 2024). In Garden State Hospital, there have been various adverse incidents involving racism towards patients of color. Such experiences compromise the quality of care offered and diminish trust in the healthcare system. Studying these cases will also help us realize that discrimination is present almost everywhere and that it is high time to make changes at the systemic level.

Among the most appalling cases of discrimination, there is a patient with epilepsy who requires the assistance of a service dog. This patient said that they experienced prejudice and aggression on the part of the hospital workers. Surprisingly, some of the staff members were allegedly discourteous and uncompliant to the presence and necessity of the service dog in handling the patient's condition. The patient reported specific instances when they were asked about the service dog's necessity and treated improperly, almost like an annoyance. Such discrimination not only created pressure but also overlapped with the patient's epilepsy care. A shortage of service animals shows that there is a significant loophole in the hospital's diversity and sensitivity policies.

One example involves an Asian patient who encountered racism when she was pregnant with her second child, which was a high-risk pregnancy. The patient recalled that the medical staff paid her less attention than others, and her voice was often ignored, giving her lesser attention as a patient. This discrimination only added to her anxiety and fear during a time that was already quite delicate. Due to the perceived disrespect and lack of attention from the healthcare provider, the patient experienced poor healthcare encounters. Such cases highlight the impact of racial prejudice in medical facilities, particularly during emergencies like high-risk pregnancies.

These individual accounts are one of the common forms of discrimination experienced by different patients at Garden State Hospital. Essays and testimonials suggest that discrimination can be expressed in various forms, from straightforward prejudiced remarks to subtle mistreatment. Minority patients understand they need to be more assertive when demanding their right to proper medical care, and this drains them emotionally.

Discrimination can also hurt health since stress and anxiety from discrimination can be detrimental to one's health and ability to recover from illnesses.

The effects of discrimination in healthcare facilities are evident from the existing literature. Research has also revealed that ethnic and racial minorities receive inferior care than white individuals, resulting in health inequalities (Odonkor et al., 2021; Zavala et al., 2021). Discrimination can make patients avoid seeking health care when they need it most, thereby causing them to suffer for a long (Meyerson et al., 2021). Healthcare providers must be trained to identify and prevent biases to produce a non-discriminatory setting.

The following strategies must be implemented to solve these shortcomings in Garden State Hospital. First, a stipulation for staff development in diversity, equity, and inclusion must be made. Such training should, in particular, address implicit bias and potential variability in patients' requirements. Second, the hospital must have unequivocal guidelines regarding treating and accommodating service animals for all patients. Third, implementing robust reporting procedures to make patients comfortable reporting discrimination cases is essential for holding them accountable and improving.

Policies and Training for Inclusivity

Garden State Hospital has implemented the following policies to ensure all patients receive equal treatment free from bias. These policies aim to respond to the different needs of the hospital's patients irrespective of their race, ethnicity, and socioeconomic status. According to its mission statement, this hospital aims to be caring and honor each person's dignity. Furthermore, the hospital has established different training sessions to raise awareness around COFL sensitivities and diversity within the health sector.

However, the efficiency of such measures still needs to be measured based on the patient experiences and testimonials. Some staff members fully understand and appreciate the importance of diversity while others do not; for instance, the aspect of addressing patients with disabilities, including those using service animals in the hospital, is not well implemented in the hospital by various staff. Such discrepancies can lead to discrimination, as evidenced by the case of a patient with epilepsy who had numerous issues due to the staff's refusal to allow the service dog. This case illustrates a significant decoupling between the formal policies in place and the actual actions taken, suggesting that more work is needed to improve the enforcement and oversight of these diversity policies.

The hospital's training on diversity is good but may need more depth and be sufficiently frequent. Training for implicit bias and cultural competence is essential for all healthcare workers, as it allows them to serve all patients with dignity and fairness. However, certain staff members may only be briefly trained, and some may not be compelled to continue polishing such issues. It can result in ignorance and insensitivity when dealing with patients from different cultural backgrounds. For instance, an Asian patient during a high-risk pregnancy expressed her feelings of discrimination and exclusion, which may indicate that staff members do not recognize the need or value of the provision of culturally sensitive care to patients from different cultural backgrounds.

However, Garden State Hospital should consider conducting broader and more frequent employee training for the above inclusivity measures to be effective. Ideally, these programs should extend beyond a simple understanding of cultural differences and include recognizing bias, prejudice, and social factors affecting health. Conducting workshops, seminars, and training sessions ensures that every worker knows the best practices for delivering inclusive care (Chu et al., 2021). Further, using case studies and patients' experiences can enhance training and make it more practical.

Moreover, the hospital must have proper procedures for monitoring and assessing the success of its inclusivity policies. This could entail conducting periodic assessments such as audits, patient satisfaction surveys, and mystery clients to determine the extent of compliance with the hospital's policies on patient-centered care for the LGBT community. It is also essential to develop clear procedures for handling discrimination concerns and guarantee that such concerns are not disregarded and are addressed effectively (Kirkland & Hyman, 2021). By ensuring its staff is always on their toes and aware of the hospital's policy towards Staffing and inclusiveness, the hospital can improve its performance and policy set.

Despite having diversity policies and training programs in place at Garden State Hospital, the implementation varies. The hospital needs to increase its training activities and set up better compliance measures to guarantee that all patients are treated fairly and respectfully. In this way, the hospital can achieve the goal of its mission statement and provide supportive care while respecting the inherent worth and value of each human being.

CASE STUDIES

The effects of prejudice at Garden State Hospital can be described based on the personal stories of some patients. One such account was of an African American patient who had a service dog for epilepsy and had been treated horribly. The patient complained of being asked numerous times about the service dog's legitimacy even after the paperwork was submitted. The workers in the hospital also failed to show compassion and respect, making the patient feel uncomfortable and neglected. This, indeed, was not only an emotional ordeal for the patient but also detrimental to the patient's well-being and health status.

One of the examples presented described a high-risk pregnancy Asian woman who felt overlooked and unappreciated by the healthcare workers. She said her complaints were disregarded, and she did not receive the same attention as other patients. This kind of discrimination made her more anxious while she was already stressed and damaged her trust in the healthcare providers. This lack of cultural differences and the appropriate approach affected her medical care experience.

Such personal accounts only prove the existence of discrimination in Garden State Hospital and the necessity of change. The stories raise awareness of how biases reduce patients' quality of care, well-being, and confidence in the healthcare system. Combating these types of discrimination requires extensive orientation and rigorous adherence to non-discrimination policies in providing patient care services.

FIVE
SYSTEMIC ISSUES AND IMPROVEMENT STRATEGIES

SYSTEMIC ISSUES IDENTIFIED

Several system problems directly affect Garden State Hospital and its patients' quality of care and organizational effectiveness. The textual analysis of patient feedback shows that patients complain about broken communication, paperwork issues, and employee disorganization. These problems affect the overall patient experience and hinder the hospital's ability to provide safe, effective care.

Among them, the main one is the need for more effective communication between patients and healthcare workers in many cases. Interpersonal communication facilitates accurate diagnosis, proper treatments, and patient satisfaction (Burgener, 2020). Nevertheless, patients often complain that they get contradicting information from one doctor to another or need more adequate information on their conditions and treatment plans or impending procedures. For instance, a patient stated how they received contradicting advice from different doctors, which left them confused and stressed about their illness. Such inconsistencies in communication lead to misdiagnosis and incorrect treatment, thereby increasing stress levels among the patients and negatively affecting their health condition.

The Garden State Hospital also needs more efficiency in its administrative systems. Several patient interviews reveal concerns like extended waiting periods, administrative formalities, and slow processing of admissions and discharges. Such inefficiencies cause much inconvenience to the patients and their families who seek a fast and efficient service (Kwame & Petrucka, 2021). Another common anecdote relates to the billing section, where patients allege that they have been charged the wrong amount and have yet to be able to resolve the problem. For example, a patient complained about paying multiple wrong bills yearly due to the hospital's inability to keep proper insurance details. Such administrative issues affect the patient and create more issues within the hospital and staff, thus adding further inconveniences and unhappiness.

Another essential problem is the need for better collaboration between different departments and healthcare organizations within the hospital. Coordination is crucial to avoid gaps in patient care, particularly for patients with multiple chronic illnesses

(Karam et al., 2021). Nevertheless, several patients have been delayed and confused at Garden State Hospital due to poor coordination. The following patient's account described a surgical procedure that involved many delays and inconsistent instructions from the surgical and nursing teams. This situation can result in medical mistakes, longer hospitalizations, and eroded confidence in the hospital's capacity to deliver integrated care.

The constant challenges of communication gaps, poor administrative practices, and poor coordination at Garden State Hospital are significant systems-level challenges that require redress to enhance the quality of care. The literature has indicated that increasing these aspects yields desirable impacts on patients' health status and satisfaction (Burgener, 2020). For example, following the set communication guidelines and the mandatory orientation of the healthcare personnel, misunderstandings may be minimized, and the information delivered more understandable for the patient. Also, reducing central-office paperwork and implementing enhanced data-handling systems help eliminate delays or confusion over billings.

To tackle these problems, a multifaceted model must include all hospital personnel, managers, and caregivers. Hence, by paying attention to voice, working on the organizational structure, and increasing collaboration between departments, Garden State Hospital can work on creating a more effective and patient-centric system. All these improvements will help the patients by delivering more accurate and empathetic care and help the hospital's management function efficiently and cost-effectively.

In conclusion, several problems influence patient experiences at Garden State Hospital, including communication challenges, hierarchy, and coordination. Solving these issues with specific measures and structural changes is necessary to enhance the hospital and patients' outcomes and ensure that every patient receives the quality care they need and deserve. Addressing these issues can help Garden State Hospital improve its standing and achieve its goal of offering outstanding care to the community.

EFFECTS ON PATIENT CONFIDENCE AND SATISFACTION

These gaps include communication breakdowns, lack of effective and efficient administration, and poor coordination between different Garden State Hospital teams, negatively impacting patients' trust and satisfaction. Trust is an essential factor in the patient-provider relationship, and if eroded, the patient will not be sticking to the doctor's prescriptions, recommendations, or appointments again (Wu et al., 2022). The recurrent issues in the hospital affect not only the discrete experiences of patients but also general conclusions about trustworthiness and effectiveness.

Interactions between doctors and patients are frequently characterized by misunderstandings that may have adverse consequences (Vermeir et al., 2015). For instance, one of the patients described a case where different doctors gave them opposing information concerning their treatment regime. This led to confusion and anxiety because the patient could not understand which of the given pieces of advice to follow. Inadequate and ambiguous information sharing left the patient needing more trust in the doctors, thus affecting their participation in the treatment plan. Those are examples of what can happen when communication becomes problematic and patient trust is lost.

Administrative inefficiencies, such as long wait times and billing discrepancies, further diminish patient satisfaction. They provided feedback on experiences, such as being billed in error, which would take months to be corrected. Even though the patient repeated the insurance details several times, she still received the bills that did not match, which created a lot of stress and financial burden for her. This left the patient feeling ignored and unappreciated, as if the hospital administration needed to care for their opinions. Such clerical mistakes cause inconvenience for patients and damage their confidence in the hospital's handling of their affairs.

An example of how systems affect patient trust is the need for integration between hospital departments. A patient described an incident where they underwent surgery in which the surgical and nursing teams were not communicating. The lack of coordination resulted in multiple delays and more precise instructions, which only frustrated the patient. The patient's faith in the hospital continued to diminish when they had to deal with these problems independently with minimal assistance or directions from the workers. This is more so when the patient is challenged with other health complications yet is on their own to manage such systemic issues.

Literature in the healthcare domain shows how these systemic issues affect patient satisfaction. Research has found that patients with poor communication, bureaucratic delays, and fragmented care feel dissatisfied and do not trust their providers (Wieke Noviyanti et al., 2021). These negative experiences may result in patients not seeking medical attention when they need to, delaying their treatment, and seeking medical attention elsewhere, worsening their health complications.

These issues stem from systemic problems that need to be resolved for Garden State Hospital to regain patients' trust and satisfaction. Standard communication procedures can enhance patient understanding to avoid miscommunication between doctors. Efficiency can be improved by training the staff on administrative procedures to minimize billing errors and the admission and discharge processes. Addressing this issue by ensuring that there is proper communication between departments can also reduce the frustration that patients go through due to such hitches.

In conclusion, the system failures at Garden State Hospital significantly affect patient trust and satisfaction. Lack of clarity, bureaucracy, and poor coordination result in poor patient health outcomes and loss of confidence in the hospital by the patient. Coping with these problems on operational, tactical, and strategic levels will help the hospital enhance patient experiences, regain their trust, and guarantee all the clients the best outcomes possible.

STRATEGIES FOR IMPROVEMENT

Thus, the identified systemic problems at Garden State Hospital require a comprehensive solution. Care delivery, coordination, and patient outcomes must be addressed through specific interventions and coordinated collective initiatives of the hospital employees. Garden State can develop a more efficient and patient-friendly healthcare system through other hospitals' current reforms and best practices.

One of the significant areas that require enhancement is communication. This implies that proper communication between healthcare providers and their patients should always be to facilitate proper diagnosis and treatment (Wu et al., 2022). Sainthe t Peter's should establish communication procedures with its departments to improve communication. This may mean having daily or weekly interdisciplinary conferences to review patient care planning and progression and utilizing EHR to guarantee that all care providers are current on the patient's status. It is also possible to organize training related to communication skills to ensure that staff members provide patients with clear and relevant information and with proper empathy.

Evidence shows that many administrative practices in Garden State Hospital must be more effective and redesigned. These can be made effective by applying principles like reducing human interference in certain processes, such as appoisuchaas rs and billing. Improving data management practices can increase the proper documentation of patient data to minimize differences in billing and decrease points of administrative bottlenecks (Verma et al., 2021). For instance, the Healthcare Financial Management Association (HFMA) reported that healthcare facilities implementing the automated billing system recorded fewer billing errors and quicker settlement of reimbursement disputes (HFMA, 2018).

Other recommendations contributing to overall patient care include embracing patient safety culture improvement and promoting accountability. This can be achieved by developing guidelines for assessing the satisfaction level of patients and handling their grievances (O'Donovan et al., 2019). For example, administering patient feedback surveys on a routine basis can generate ideas about areas of improvement and monitor the success of change processes (Kirkland & Hyman, 2021). Also, implementing the best practices and guidelines will guarantee all patients receive equal quality health care services. For example, implementing care bundles, which are collections of interventions shown to enhance patient outcomes, can reduce variability in patient care through bundles of practices.

Examples from similar hospitals can be used as information and inspiration when implementing change at Garden State Hospital. An example is the Cleveland Clinic, which has received awards for patient care innovations and effective operations. Cleveland Clinic built a patient experience program with intensive staff education, continuous gathering of feedback from patients, and an emphasis on communication and compassion (Mustafa et al., 2019). This has enhanced patient satisfaction levels and the general quality of care offered in the hospital.

Another example is Intermountain Healthcare, which, to date, has overcome several administrative hurdles and enhanced patient care quality by adopting integrated care management information systems. With an integrative approach to patient management and the applied use of innovative tools to optimize administrative work, Intermountain Healthcare has improved patient outcomes and evaluation scores (Ostler, 2022). These examples show that implementing a systems-based, tailored approach to delivering patient care might have certain advantages.

Better billing practices are necessary to counter the problem of billing discrepancies in Garden State Hospital. This may involve implementing fully automated billing systems that prevent human intervention and promote efficient insurance data management (Cooper et al., 2020). Other mitigation steps include ensuring that the billing and coding staff is trained on the best practices to avoid errors. Developing a separate group to address the patients' billing concerns and complaints would help patients trust that their billing concerns would be addressed early and adequately.

Another part of the improvement strategy is, for example, enhanced staff training programs. Consistency in training sessions on cultural sensitivity, perceived bias, and patient interactions may assist the staff in delivering culturally sensitive and patient-centered care (Stubbe et al., 2020). For instance, it may be possible to adopt simulation-based training activities that would help prepare the staff to handle such sensitive issues and patients.

AFTERWORD

Throughout this book, we have explored numerous facets of patient experiences at Garden State Hospital and found countless positive aspects as well as shortcomings. The main conclusions based on such investigation refer to systematic problems such as ineffective communication, mismanagement of bureaucratic tasks, and the absence of collaboration among the hospital's employees. These recurrent issues have significant implications for patient confidence and perceptions of care, highlighting the urgent and essential requirement for systemic changes.

One of the main issues identified is the inconsistency in patient-doctor communication. Some patients received helpful and prompt answers from doctors, while others received contradictory information and poor communication that caused confusion and stress. This loses the patients' trust due to multiple billing mistakes, delayed appointments, and poor quality of service delivery. These problems are made worse by poor departmental integration, whereby patient care gets delayed, and patients receive more precise instructions and decisions from the different departments.

However, it is equally important to look at Garden State Hospital's strengths, and here they are. Some patients have commended the hospital for the medical staff's kind nature and hard work. When systems are optimized, positive experiences, particularly in specific sectors such as oncology, prove that the medical institution can provide adequate care. However, broader organizational factors often overshadow such positive experiences that negatively impact patient satisfaction.

Thus, our findings' implications apply to Garden State Hospital and are generalizable to the healthcare organization. The problems described here are not exclusive to this particular hospital; they are typical for most hospitals. Resolving these issues is crucial to enhancing the quality of healthcare delivery and guaranteeing that all clients are offered the quality and sensitive care they require. This can be completed simply by having good communication, efficient business practices, and integrated health care.

Making healthcare better can only happen if there is value placed in learning and change. Organizations must ensure staff undergo adequate orientation and adhere to formal procedures for reaching out to others and supporting patients. Thus, promoting a culture of accountability and patient-centered care can help restore trust and enhance outcomes in healthcare institutions. The information drawn from the patient's feedback and experiences shared in their narratives is useful to inform these efforts.

The aim of writing this book is to provide further discourses on the improvement of healthcare services. By addressing some of the issues Garden State Hospital patients face, we would like to raise awareness of the existing problems and possible solutions in the modern health delivery process. Patient feedback is an effective way of learning where changes need to be made, thus making it possible to create more positive changes. We urge Garden State Hospital to consider these findings and make the desired changes to improve patient experiences.

Altogether, approaching the problems at Garden State Hospital on an organizational level will be the key to regaining the patients' confidence and increasing satisfaction rates. Enhancing communication, administration, and general cooperation will assist the hospital in improving workflow and its approach to patient care. The stories and comments I documented in this book serve as a blueprint that the hospital needs to emulate towards achieving its goal of being a world-class healthcare institution. With such commitment and improvement, Garden State Hospital will be able to accomplish its mission of offering comprehensive, compassionate care to all its patients.

BIBLIOGRAPHY

Åhlin, P., Almström, P., & Wänström, C. (2022). When patients get stuck: a systematic literature review on throughput barriers in hospital-wide patient processes. *Health Policy, 126*(2), 87-98.

Ahmad, I. A., & Osei, E. (2023). Occupational health and safety measures in healthcare settings during COVID-19: Strategies for protecting staff, patients, and visitors. *Disaster Medicine and Public Health Preparedness, 17*, e48.

Asamrew, N., Endris, A. A., & Tadesse, M. (2020). Level of patient satisfaction with inpatient services and its determinants: a study of a specialized hospital in Ethiopia. *Journal of environmental and public health, 2020*(1), 2473469.

Bhati, D., Deogade, M. S., & Kanyal, D. (2023). Improving Patient Outcomes Through Effective Hospital Administration: A Comprehensive Review. *Cureus, 15*(10), e47731. https://doi.org/10.7759/cureus.47731

Boissy, A., Windover, A. K., Bokar, D., Karafa, M., Neuendorf, K., Frankel, R. M., Merlino, J., & Rothberg, M. B. (2016). Communication Skills Training for Physicians Improves Patient Satisfaction. *Journal of general internal medicine, 31*(7), 755–761. https://doi.org/10.1007/s11606-016-3597-2

Browne, K., & Mitchell, B. G. (2023). Multimodal environmental cleaning strategies to prevent healthcare-associated infections. *Antimicrobial resistance and infection control, 12*(1), 83. https://doi.org/10.1186/s13756-023-01274-4

Buljac-Samardzic, M., Doekhie, K. D., & van Wijngaarden, J. D. (2020). Interventions to improve team effectiveness within health care: a systematic review of the past decade. *Human resources for health, 18*, 1-42.

Burgener, A. M. (2020). Enhancing communication to improve patient safety and to increase patient satisfaction. *The health care manager, 39*(3), 128-132.

Chu, C. H., McGilton, K. S., Spilsbury, K., Le, K. N., Boscart, V., Backman, A., ... & Zúñiga, F. (2021). Strengthening international research in long-term care: recommended common data elements to support clinical staff training. *Gerontology and Geriatric Medicine, 7*, 2333721421999312.

Cooper, Z., Nguyen, H., Shekita, N., & Morton, F. S. (2020). Out-Of-Network Billing And Negotiated Payments For Hospital-Based Physicians: The cost impact of specialists who bill patients at out-of-network rates even though the patients do not choose and cannot avoid these specialists, such as anesthesiologists. *Health Affairs, 39*(1), 24-32.

Damery, S., Flanagan, S., Jones, J., & Jolly, K. (2021). The Effect of Providing Staff Training and Enhanced Support to Care Homes on Care Processes, Safety Climate and Avoidable Harms: Evaluation of a Care Home Quality Improvement Programme in England. *International journal of environmental research and public health, 18*(14), 7581. https://doi.org/10.3390/ijerph18147581

De Brún, A., Anjara, S., Cunningham, U., Khurshid, Z., Macdonald, S., O'Donovan, R., ... & McAuliffe, E. (2020). The collective leadership for safety culture (co-lead) team intervention to promote teamwork and patient safety. *International Journal of Environmental Research and Public Health, 17*(22), 8673.

Drossman, D. A., & Ruddy, J. (2020). Improving patient-provider relationships to improve health care. *Clinical Gastroenterology and Hepatology, 18*(7), 1417-1426.

Ferreira, D. C., Vieira, I., Pedro, M. I., Caldas, P., & Varela, M. (2023). Patient Satisfaction with Healthcare Services and the Techniques Used for its Assessment: A Systematic Literature Review and a Bibliometric Analysis. *Healthcare (Basel, Switzerland), 11*(5), 639. https://doi.org/10.3390/healthcare11050639

Flodgren, G., Gonçalves-Bradley, D. C., & Pomey, M. P. (2016). External inspection of compliance with standards for improved healthcare outcomes. *The Cochrane database of systematic reviews, 12*(12), CD008992. https://doi.org/10.1002/14651858.CD008992.pub3

Gagliardi, A. R., Yip, C. Y., Irish, J., Wright, F. C., Rubin, B., Ross, H., ... & Stewart, D. E. (2021). The psychological burden of waiting for procedures and patient-centred strategies that could support the mental health of wait-listed patients and caregivers during the COVID-19 pandemic: A scoping review. *Health Expectations*, 24(3), 978-990.

Han, S., Xu, M., Lao, J., & Liang, Z. (2023). Collecting Patient Feedback as a Means of Monitoring Patient Experience and Hospital Service Quality - Learning from a Government-led Initiative. *Patient preference and adherence, 17,* 385–400. https://doi.org/10.2147/PPA.S397444

Haque, M., McKimm, J., Sartelli, M., Dhingra, S., Labricciosa, F. M., Islam, S., ... & Charan, J. (2020). Strategies to prevent healthcare-associated infections: a narrative overview. *Risk management and healthcare policy*, 1765-1780.

Heinrich, C. J., Camacho, S., Henderson, S. C., Hernández, M., & Joshi, E. (2022). Consequences of administrative burden for social safety nets that support the healthy development of children. *Journal of Policy Analysis and Management*, 41(1), 11-44.

Jankelová, N., & Joniaková, Z. (2021). Communication Skills and Transformational Leadership Style of First-Line Nurse Managers in Relation to Job Satisfaction of Nurses and Moderators of This Relationship. *Healthcare (Basel, Switzerland)*, 9(3), 346. https://doi.org/10.3390/healthcare9030346

Jones, S., Moulton, C., Swift, S., Molyneux, P., Black, S., Mason, N., ... & Mann, C. (2022). Association between delays to patient admission from the emergency department and all-cause 30-day mortality. *Emergency Medicine Journal*, 39(3), 168-173.

Kalouguina, V., & Wagner, J. (2020). Challenges and solutions for integrating and financing personalized medicine in healthcare systems: A systematic literature review. *Journal of Risk and Financial Management*, 13(11), 283.

Karam, M., Chouinard, M. C., Poitras, M. E., Couturier, Y., Vedel, I., Grgurevic, N., & Hudon, C. (2021). Nursing care coordination for patients with complex needs in primary healthcare: a scoping review. *International Journal of Integrated Care*, 21(1).

Keshavarzi, M. H., Safaie, S., Faghihi, S. A. A., & Zare, S. (2022). Barriers of physician-patient relationships in professionalism: A qualitative study. *Journal of advances in medical education &*

professionalism, 10(3), 199–206. https://doi.org/10.30476/JAMP.2022.94010.1563

Kirkland, A., & Hyman, M. (2021). Civil rights as patient experience: How healthcare organizations handle discrimination complaints. *Law & Society Review, 55*(2), 273-295.

Kwame, A., & Petrucka, P. M. (2021). A literature-based study of patient-centered care and communication in nurse-patient interactions: barriers, facilitators, and the way forward. *BMC nursing, 20*(1), 158. https://doi.org/10.1186/s12912-021-00684-2

Lindström, V., Sturesson, L., & Carlborg, A. (2020). Patients' experiences of the caring encounter with the psychiatric emergency response team in the emergency medical service—A qualitative interview study. *Health Expectations, 23*(2), 442-449.

Liu, Q., Luo, D., Haase, J. E., Guo, Q., Wang, X. Q., Liu, S., ... & Yang, B. X. (2020). The experiences of healthcare providers during the COVID-19 crisis in China: a qualitative study. *The Lancet Global Health, 8*(6), e790-e798.

Magnusson, C., Herlitz, J., & Axelsson, C. (2020). Patient characteristics, triage utilisation, level of care, and outcomes in an unselected adult patient population seen by the emergency medical services: a prospective observational study. *BMC Emergency Medicine, 20*, 1-19.

Mahmoudi, E., Kamdar, N., Kim, N., Gonzales, G., Singh, K., & Waljee, A. K. (2020). Use of electronic medical records in development and validation of risk prediction models of hospital readmission: systematic review. *bmj, 369*.

Maki, G., & Zervos, M. (2021). Health care–acquired infections in low- and middle-income countries and the role of infection prevention and control. *Infectious Disease Clinics, 35*(3), 827-839.

Marca-Frances, G., Frigola-Reig, J., Menéndez-Signorini, J. A., Compte-Pujol, M., & Massana-Morera, E. (2020). Defining patient communication needs during hospitalization to improve patient experience and health literacy. *BMC health services research, 20*, 1-9.

Meyerson, B. E., Russell, D. M., Kichler, M., Atkin, T., Fox, G., & Coles, H. B. (2021). I don't even want to go to the doctor when I get sick now: healthcare experiences and discrimination reported by people who use drugs, Arizona 2019. *International Journal of Drug Policy, 93*, 103112.

BIBLIOGRAPHY

Mustafa, S., Farver, C. F., Bierer, S. B., & Stoller, J. K. (2019). Impact of a leadership development program for healthcare executives: the Cleveland Clinic experience. *Journal of Health Administration Education*, 36(1), 77-91.

Noble, L. M. (2020). Doctor-patient communication and adherence to treatment. In *Adherance to Treatment in Medical Conditions* (pp. 51-82). CRC Press.

O'Donovan, R., Ward, M., De Brún, A., & McAuliffe, E. (2019). Safety culture in health care teams: A narrative review of the literature. *Journal of nursing management*, 27(5), 871-883.

Odonkor, C. A., Esparza, R., Flores, L. E., Verduzco–Gutierrez, M., Escalon, M. X., Solinsky, R., & Silver, J. K. (2021). Disparities in health care for black patients in physical medicine and rehabilitation in the United States: a narrative review. *PM&R*, 13(2), 180-203.

Ostler, C. R. (2022). *Intermountain Healthcare: Utilizing Technology to Bring Value to Patients*. SAGE Publications: SAGE Business Cases Originals.

Peters, A., Schmid, M. N., Parneix, P., Lebowitz, D., de Kraker, M., Sauser, J., ... & Pittet, D. (2022). Impact of environmental hygiene interventions on healthcare-associated infections and patient colonization: a systematic review. *Antimicrobial Resistance & Infection Control*, 11(1), 38.

Prakash, G., & Srivastava, S. (2020). Exploring value-dense environment in the healthcare service delivery: a patient-centric perspective. *The TQM Journal*, 32(2), 331-347.

Prakitsuwan, P., & Promsit, S. (2022). *Embracing service design for hospital patient-centred experience: case study in health check-up centre* (Doctoral dissertation, Thammasat University).

Rodziewicz, T. L., & Hipskind, J. E. (2020). Medical error prevention. *StatPearls. Treasure Island (FL): StatPearls Publishing*.

Garden State Healthcare System. (n.d.). About us. Retrieved June 17, 2024, from https://www.saintpetershcs.com/about-us

Sharma, S., Kaushik, V., & Tiwari, V. (2023). Role of biofilms in hospital-acquired infections (HAIs). In *Understanding Microbial Biofilms* (pp. 209-245). Academic Press.

Singh, G., Patel, R. H., Vaqar, S., & Boster, J. (2024). Root cause analysis and medical error prevention. In *StatPearls [internet]*. StatPearls Publishing.

Singh, H., & Dey, A. K. (2021). Listen to my story: Contribution of patients to their healthcare through effective communication with doctors. *Health Services Management Research*, 34(3), 178-192.

Smith C. P. (2017). First, do no harm: institutional betrayal and trust in health care organizations. *Journal of multidisciplinary healthcare*, 10, 133–144. https://doi.org/10.2147/JMDH.S125885

Stangl, A. L., Earnshaw, V. A., Logie, C. H., van Brakel, W., C Simbayi, L., Barré, I., & Dovidio, J. F. (2019). The Health Stigma and Discrimination Framework: a global, crosscutting framework to inform research, intervention development, and policy on health-related stigmas. *BMC medicine*, 17(1), 31. https://doi.org/10.1186/s12916-019-1271-3

Steinmair, D., Zervos, K., Wong, G., & Löffler-Stastka, H. (2022). Importance of communication in medical practice and medical education: an emphasis on empathy and attitudes and their possible influences. *World Journal of Psychiatry*, 12(2), 323.

Stubbe D. E. (2020). Practicing Cultural Competence and Cultural Humility in the Care of Diverse Patients. *Focus (American Psychiatric Publishing)*, 18(1), 49–51. https://doi.org/10.1176/appi.focus.20190041

Tavakoly Sany, S. B., Behzhad, F., Ferns, G., & Peyman, N. (2020). Communication skills training for physicians improves health literacy and medical outcomes among patients with hypertension: a randomized controlled trial. *BMC health services research*, 20, 1-10.

Togioka, B., Duvivier, D., & Young, E. (2024). Diversity and Discrimination in Health Care. *StatPearls*.

Umuhoza, A. G., Kamugisha, J. B., Nashwan, A. J., & Soko, G. T. (2023). Assessment of knowledge and practices of hand hygiene among health workers in Rwanda. *International Journal of Africa Nursing Sciences*, 19, 100585.

van Hout, D., Hutchinson, P., Wanat, M., Pilbeam, C., Goossens, H., Anthierens, S., ... & Gobat, N. (2022). The experience of European hospital-based health care workers on following infection prevention and control procedures and their well-being during the first wave of the COVID-19 pandemic. *PLoS One*, 17(2), e0245182.

BIBLIOGRAPHY

Verma, A. A., Pasricha, S. V., Jung, H. Y., Kushnir, V., Mak, D. Y., Koppula, R., ... & Razak, F. (2021). Assessing the quality of clinical and administrative data extracted from hospitals: the General Medicine Inpatient Initiative (GEMINI) experience. *Journal of the American Medical Informatics Association, 28*(3), 578-587.

Vermeir, P., Vandijck, D., Degroote, S., Peleman, R., Verhaeghe, R., Mortier, E., Hallaert, G., Van Daele, S., Buylaert, W., & Vogelaers, D. (2015). Communication in healthcare: a narrative review of the literature and practical recommendations. *International journal of clinical practice, 69*(11), 1257–1267. https://doi.org/10.1111/ijcp.12686

Wieke Noviyanti, L., Ahsan, A., & Sudartya, T. S. (2021). Exploring the relationship between nurses' communication satisfaction and patient safety culture. *Journal of public health research, 10*(2), 2225. https://doi.org/10.4081/jphr.2021.2225

Wu, D., Lowry, P. B., Zhang, D., & Tao, Y. (2022). Patient Trust in Physicians Matters-Understanding the Role of a Mobile Patient Education System and Patient-Physician Communication in Improving Patient Adherence Behavior: Field Study. *Journal of medical Internet research, 24*(12), e42941. https://doi.org/10.2196/42941

Zavala, V. A., Bracci, P. M., Carethers, J. M., Carvajal-Carmona, L., Coggins, N. B., Cruz-Correa, M. R., ... & Fejerman, L. (2021). Cancer health disparities in racial/ethnic minorities in the United States. *British journal of cancer, 124*(2), 315-332.

Zepeda-Lugo, C., Tlapa, D., Baez-Lopez, Y., Limon-Romero, J., Ontiveros, S., Perez-Sanchez, A., & Tortorella, G. (2020). Assessing the Impact of Lean Healthcare on Inpatient Care: A Systematic Review. *International journal of environmental research and public health, 17*(15), 5609. https://doi.org/10.3390/ijerph17155609

Printed in the USA
CPSIA information can be obtained
at www.ICGtesting.com
LVHW021207191124
797036LV00013B/499